# Table of Contents

# Copyright

# Introduction

I want to thank you and congratulate you for downloading the book, *"Fermentation: Fermentation for Beginners, Fermentation Recipes rich in Probiotics, Enzymes, Vitamins, Minerals - LEARN To Ferment Foods Now"*.

This book contains useful information on how to start fermenting your own food.

You may feel intimidated by the whole fermentation process. But this book will show you that fermenting your own vegetables and fruits can be an enjoyable and rewarding experience. You will benefit from eating flavorful food that is also downright healthy.

Hopefully, this book will help you learn exactly why probiotics, enzymes, vitamins, and minerals are good for your health and encourage you to enjoy eating more healthy food.

Thanks again for downloading this book, I hope you enjoy it!

# Chapter 1: Guidelines to Fermenting Food

## The Health Benefits of Fermented Foods

### Rediscover Healthy Food

On one hand, if you are not fond of eating vegetables, fruits, and milk, eating fermented food will let you enjoy them for the first time and get you hooked to eating healthy food for life.

On the other hand, if dairy, fruits, and vegetables have always been part of your diet, but then you have been eating them out of duty and not because you love how they taste, then fermented food will be your ticket to eating them with gusto.

### Spend Less on All-natural Vitamins and Minerals

Your body will benefit from the vitamins and minerals that are naturally present in vegetables, fruits, and milk. These plant-based nutrients are infinitely better than the ones available in synthetic supplements, which are too expensive for anyone's taste, but are not necessarily absorbed by your body effectively.

### Enjoy Your Milk to the Fullest

You will also have your share of the healthy goodness of enzymes (special proteins that help your body enhance its processes). Fermentation breaks down the enzymes found in milk and milk products to let your body absorb them better.

## Arm Your Gut with the Power of Probiotics

Fermenting your food lets your stomach get back the optimal number of good bacteria needed to keep it healthy. Probiotics are your body's natural defense against harmful microorganisms that inevitably enter your stomach when eating certain food that you did not prepare yourself. In restaurants, some food may unknowingly be prepared in less than sanitary conditions. During parties, some food may not have been cooked thoroughly by the host who may have been pressed for time.

# The Principles of Fermentation

## Simple Way of Preparing Healthy Food

Seriously, there is no faster way of killing one's appetite for healthy eating than the thought of preparing it! Cooking vegetables take too much time. And all the peeling, cutting, coring, and juicing involved in preparing your fruits are enough to want you to eliminate them from your diet altogether. Fermentation lets you enjoy your fruits and vegetables in a lazy manner because there is no cooking involved (yay!).

## Easy on the Budget

The advantage of preparing fermented food is not just the small amount of time it requires you to give, but the tools you need could be had without burning a hole in your pocket.

## Brings Back the Joy in Cooking

You can't help but have fun in the kitchen while you are whipping up different fermented food. You only need the most basic tools – whey (to start the fermentation process), fermenting jars, chopping board, knife, and your clean hands. The most tasking part involved in fermenting food is simply checking up on them during the fermentation period, and that is just to make sure they are still submerged under their juices. What could be easier than that?

# Chapter 2: Recipes - Fermented Vegetable Salads

## Easiest Sauerkraut on Earth

*Also known as "sour cabbage" as well as a rich source of vitamins and probiotics, sauerkraut is a popular fermented food that is surprisingly easy to make – even for a beginner like you!*

### What You Need:
How do you define easy? Easy means getting yourself a medium head of good old cabbage and some sea salt (1 to 3 tablespoons should do).

### How to Make:
Shred the cabbage you've got onto a large mixing bowl and then drizzle with salt. You may need to knead the cabbage pieces for ten minutes to get their liquid out, or you can use your trusted potato masher. The important thing is to be sure that you produce enough liquid to cover the cabbage.

Transfer the cabbage and liquid into a half-gallon fermenting jar. Because making sauerkraut calls for completely covering the cabbage pieces with liquid, it helps to add a small amount of water.
Place your cabbage-filled fermenting jar anywhere in your house that has a room temperature hovering between 60°F and 70°F. You will need to culture sauerkraut for a few days

until you get your preferred texture and flavor so it truly helps to check its quality daily. Doing so also helps to release pressure from inside the jar due to the gases naturally produced during fermentation.

When your sauerkraut is finally done fermenting at room temperature, it is time to park it inside the refrigerator, where it will go on fermenting and taste even better as it ages.
*Easy!*

# Salsa Bonanza

*Tacos and salads level up in their goodness once you complement them with this spicy salsa that gives them just the right tangy kick!*

## What You Need:

For this recipe, you will need 12 onions (preferably green), 1 ½ teaspoon of flaked red pepper, 1 ½ cup of chopped bell pepper bits, 12 medium-sized tomatoes, minced bits of 5 garlic cloves and ¾ cup of cilantro, 2 ½ tablespoons of your favorite sea salt, and the juice of one lemon.

## How to Make:

Slice the green onions and tomatoes into cubes. Place in a medium-sized bowl and add in the bits of cilantro, bell pepper, and garlic. Next, toss in the red pepper flakes, salt, and lemon juice, and then mix well.

Transfer the tossed mixture into a half-gallon fermenting jar. Depending on the temperature of the room you may park this salsa in, the fermentation process for this recipe should take 2 to 6 days. Once the salsa is done, you may keep it in the fermenting jar or transfer it to another container, as long as it is placed in the refrigerator. *Andale!*

# Quickie Kimchi with Miso

*Though this kimchi leans more towards being traditional, the quick way with which you can do this surely spells modern!*

**What You Need:**
This recipe calls for the following: 2 tablespoons of rice flour (preferably the sweet variety), 3 pieces of green onions, peeled pieces of 4 garlic cloves, 2 tablespoons of fish sauce (choose one that is preservative-free), and 2 tablespoons of sugar.

You will also need ¼ cup of sea salt, 1 ¼ cup of filtered water, peeled bits of 1 inch piece of ginger, 3 tablespoons of miso, 2 large heads of cabbage, and anywhere from 2 to 8 pieces of red chili peppers to suit your desired amount of heat.

**How to Make:**
To prepare the salted cabbage, chop the heads roughly, place in a large mixing bowl, and then set aside for half an hour after tossing in the salt. Make sure to stir the cabbage-and-salt mixture after the first 15 minutes.

In making the rice flour paste, start by combining the sweet rice flour and filtered water in a separate bowl, whisking, and then heating the mixture until it reaches the boiling point. Stir the mixture continuously for a few minutes, and then let it cool.

Put on gloves before preparing the peppers. Remove the stems, seeds, and/or inner membrane with a slotted spoon. The more parts you remove, the milder your kimchi will turn out. Place the pepper as well as the remaining ingredients in your trusty food processor and blend away. After all the ingredients are chopped, add in the rice flour paste and blend again until the whole mixture becomes smooth.

Now, it is time to bring them all together! Go back to your salted cabbage and squeeze thoroughly before placing in another bowl. Pour in the seasoned rice flour paste and mix well with your gloved hands.

Place the whole mixture in a half-gallon fermenting jar and let fermentation do its job for at least 7 days. Check the mixture every once in a while, making sure that the cabbage is submerged under the brine produced everyday.

After the fermentation period, store your salsa in the refrigerator where it can continue fermenting to enhance its flavor.
*Splendid!*

# Royal Pea Salad with Bacon and Crème Fraiche

*Meaty, creamy, and fresh... this salad is so rich, it's no wonder no princess worth her pea can possibly pass it up!*

**What You Need:**
All you will need to whip up this recipe are the following: 1/3 cup of crème fraiche, some salt and pepper to taste, the zest of half a piece of lemon, chopped pieces of one bunch of scallions, 4 ounces of thickly-sliced bacon (avoid the maple variant), and 2 pounds of frozen peas.

**How to Make:**
Boil the peas to cook until they are tender enough, and then set aside to allow them to cool to room temperature.

Using a cast-iron skillet, fry the bacon slices over low to medium heat, depending on how crispy you want them. Next, take the bacon out of the skillet to cool and drain on some paper towels. Using the oil from the fried bacon, cook the scallions for 2 minutes and cool and drain the same way as the bacon.

In a medium-sized mixing bowl, combine the cooled peas, bacon, and scallions. Toss in the crème fraiche as well as the pepper, salt, and lemon zest. Serve immediately, or store in an attractive Mason jar to keep in the refrigerator.

# Honey-sweet Sauerkraut

*This healthy salad is the perfect antidote to braving the long winter season – or to refresh yourself in the summer days – with its wonderful combination of tangy and sweet flavors!*

## What You Need:
A recipe this tasty calls for 1/3 cup of your favorite brand of apple cider vinegar, 1 teaspoon of mustard seeds, 2 cups of chopped celery, 1 cup of grated carrot, and about 4 cups of drained sauerkraut. You will also need some sea salt to taste, 2/3 cup of olive oil, and ¼ cup of chopped onion. And don't forget to add ½ cup of honey!

## How to Make:
In a large mixing bowl, mix the mustard seeds, carrots, onion, sauerkraut, and celery and then set aside.

In a smaller bowl, make your dressing by combining honey with vinegar and olive oil.

Toss the dressing into the vegetables-and-sauerkraut mixture, and then transfer the lot into a quart-sized fermenting jar. Let it ferment overnight in the refrigerator, and serve it with some sea salt to taste the next day.
*Yummy!*

# Spicy and Creamy Red Potatoes

*It's hard to believe that something so deliciously complex in its flavors could require only a few minutes of your time!*

## What You Need:
This recipe calls for the following: ¾ cup of crème fraiche, some black pepper, 3 pounds worth of quartered red potatoes, ¼ cup of chopped green onion, some basil, about 3 tablespoons of butter, 2 cloves worth of minced garlic, and some sea salt to taste.

## How to Make:
Place the red potatoes in a pot with just enough water to cover them. Boil for 20 minutes or until they feel tender enough when gently pierced with a fork. After draining the potatoes, place in a large bowl and mix in the butter. Apply a bit of mashing action on the butter-and-potatoes mixture to achieve a chunky texture.

Mix the sea salt, minced garlic, chopped green onion, and basil together and then add into the buttered potatoes. Blend everything well as you carefully pour in the crème fraiche. Lastly, place on your favorite platter and sprinkle on the black pepper to serve while it's warm.
*Delish!*

# Kraut with a Touch of Jalapeno

*Altogether crunchy, spicy, tangy, and healthy... what more could you ask from this sauerkraut with a twist? Some tacos!*

## What You Need:
This recipe calls for 1 large bunch of cilantro, 1 piece of jalapeno with the seeds removed, 2 bunches of green onions, 1/2 teaspoon of cumin, 4 tablespoons each of sea salt and garlic powder, and 2 medium-sized heads of cabbage.

## How to Make:
Work on the cabbage heads by shredding them into a large mixing bowl. Chop the jalapeno, cumin, cilantro, garlic, and green onions and mix all of them into the shredded cabbage.

Add in your sea salt before mixing them all together with your washed hands to incorporate the salt well. Spend the next 5 minutes pounding the mixture to coax the juices out of the cabbage. Place the cabbage mixture in a half-gallon fermenting jar, taking to press inside to submerge the cabbage in its own juice. Leave it at room temperature (preferably 65°F) and let it ferment for about a week. You can immediately enjoy eating some of your kraut and keep the rest in cold storage, where they can ferment more and become even more flavorful.
*Scrumptious!*

# Chapter 3 Recipes for Fermented Fruit Salads

## Probiotic Waldorf Salad

*Who knew an elegant fruit salad could still benefit from a smart upgrade with a healthy dose of good microorganisms!*

**What You Need:**
Some lettuce leaves are called for to serve this fruit salad on a platter.
You will also need ½ cup of chopped walnuts, 2 tablespoons of lemon juice, ½ cup of halved purple grapes, ½ cup of your milk kefir, diced pieces of 4 red apples, 1 cup of chopped celery, and some pepper and sea salt.

**How to Make:**
In a medium-sized mixing bowl, bring the chopped celery, red apples, purple grapes, and chopped walnuts together and mix well. In a separate bowl, combine your milk kefir and lemon juice and then toss into the fruit mixture. Mix well to coat the fruits with the milk kefir-and-lemon dressing. Add the pepper and salt and then serve on your lettuce-covered fruit platter.
*Nom nom!*

# Peach and Pecan Chutney

*Its medley of mouthwatering flavors will leave you hankering for more!*

**What You Need:**
This fruity recipe calls for 2 cups of your favorite brand of raisins, 4 fresh hot peppers, 2 cups of chopped pecans, 2 ½ tablespoons of sea salt, the juice of 5 lemons, chopped bits of 4 onions, coarsely chopped pieces of 16 pears, and 4 tablespoons of grated fresh ginger.

**How to Make:**
In a large mixing bowl, toss the chopped pears well with the pecans, hot peppers, lemon juice, raisins, onions, sea salt, and ginger. Place the mixture in a quart-sized fermenting jar and then gently press the ingredients to get the juices released. In case the extracted liquid does not fully cover the mixture, add some brine with a 1:2 sea salt and water ratio.

Park the fermenting jar in an area that has a room temperature that is slightly warmer than usual. Your chutney should be fermented and good to eat after 2 to 4 days. Check on it during the fermentation process to make sure the mixture is constantly submerged under the juices. Once done, you can easily transfer the chutney in the refrigerator.
  *Refreshing!*

# Milky Orange Salad

*Refreshing and rich at the same time, this fruit salad is a tempting feast for the eyes!*

**What You Need:**
This easy recipe only calls for 3 tablespoons of chopped pistachios, ½ cup of milk kefir, a splash of vanilla extract, 1 tablespoon of honey, and 2 large oranges.

**How to Make:**
Separate the oranges into its segments, chop into bite-sized chunks, remove the seeds, and then transfer in a small bowl. Set aside to work on your dressing.

In a pint-sized fermenting jar, mix the honey, milk kefir, and vanilla by putting on the lid and shaking vigorously. Pour this dressing over the orange segments and then put in the refrigerator for about 30 minutes to give all of the flavors some time to blend together.

When ready to serve, sprinkle the chopped pistachios over the chilled and well-blended fruit salad.
*Juicy!*

# Savory Apple Salad

*There is only one way to describe this salad – easy! And it tastes great, too!*

## What You Need:
This simple recipe calls for 1 teaspoon of apple cider vinegar, minced bits of 2 garlic cloves, a pinch of ground cumin, ½ cup of milk kefir, quartered slices of 2 large apples, and ½ teaspoon of sea salt.

## How to Make:
Mix the apple cider vinegar, garlic, cumin, and milk kefir in a medium-sized bowl. Stir the dressing well before adding in the apple slices. Toss to coat the apples thoroughly and then chill in the refrigerator for 10 to 15 minutes before serving. Sprinkle on the sea salt to taste before serving.
*Done!*

# Minty Cantaloupe Salad

*You can serve this cool and creamy salad both as a dessert and as an accompaniment to a hearty breakfast of bacon and eggs!*

## What You Need:
For this recipe, you will need 2 large bananas, 1 ½ teaspoons of dried spearmint, a pinch of salt, 2 medium-sized apples, 1 ½ cups of milk kefir, 2 teaspoons of lemon juice, and 1 large cantaloupe.

## How to Make:
Chop the bananas, apples, and cantaloupes into bite-size chunks, toss altogether in a large mixing bowl, and set aside.

To make the dressing, combine your milk kefir, mint, lemon juice, and sea salt in a smaller bowl. Mix well and pour over the fruit mixture to coat. Place in the refrigerator for about 15 minutes before serving this delicious salad.
*Delightful!*

# Tangy Pina Colada Fruit Salad

*Fresh and sweet, you'll enjoy this salad's tangy twist!*

## What You Need:
For this recipe, you will need ¼ cup of coconut milk, 1-inch slices of 2 medium-sized pineapples, 3 tablespoons of honey, 1 cup of unsweetened coconut flakes, ½-inch slices of 2 bananas, and 1 ½ cups of milk kefir.

## How to Make:
In a large mixing bowl, combine the banana and pineapple slices. Add in the coconut flakes and toss. Next, make the coconut-milk honey dressing by warming the two ingredients over low heat for about 2 minutes. Then pour over the mixture of fruits and coconut flakes. Toss well to coat the fruits and refrigerate for at least 30 minutes before serving with a sprinkle of leftover coconut flakes (if there is some).
*Tasty!*

# Chapter 4 Recipes for Fermented Beverages

## Easy Water Kefir

*This simple beverage lets you have your share of fizziness and probiotics!*

### What You Need:
For this recipe, you will need ¼ cup of water kefir grains, 2 pieces of a halved lemon, ¼ cup of organic cane sugar, and 2 pieces of dried figs (unsulphured).

### How to Make:
Prepare the sugar water by heating 6 cups of filtered water. After 10 minutes, add in the sugar and stir. Remove from heat and continue stirring until the sugar completely dissolves and then let it cool to room temperature.

Place the cooled sugar water in a 2-quart fermenting jar, and then toss in the lemon halves and figs. Let the water kefir undergo fermentation for 3 days or longer, depending on how strong you would prefer the flavor to become. Once your water kefir has reached the flavor intensity you desire, transfer it to a pitcher by passing it through a strainer. Chill in the refrigerator for 15 minutes, and then serve.

# Family Milk Kefir

*If you're looking for the perfect beverage that your whole family can enjoy together – tart for Mom, effervescent for Dad, and milky for the kids - this probiotic milk drink that is high in lactobacilli and bifidus bacteria will suit you to a T!*

## What You Need:
For this recipe, all you need to work with are 4 cups of cow's milk (think fresh!) and about 2 teaspoons of milk kefir grains.

## How to Make:
Mix the two ingredients in a fermenting pint jar. To start the fermentation process, place the jar in a warm area in your kitchen; a temperature between 68° and 85°F should suffice. You only need to let 24 hours go by before culturing gets done. You'll find your milk kefir has taken on a slightly thick texture and which sets off a pleasant aroma.

Before you start drinking, separate the kefir grains from the liquid and place in another jar. This should serve you well with the next batch of milk you might wish to ferment. The remaining finished milk kefir is now ready for the taking. *Enjoy!*

# Fizzy Lemonade

*You won't be able to resist this beverage... it has refreshing written all over it!*

## What You Need:
This recipe calls for ½ cup of whey, the juice of 6 lemons, ½ cup of cane sugar, and enough filtered water to fill a half-gallon fermenting jar.

## How to Make:
Fill the fermentation jar with 2 cups of filtered water. Stir in the whey, sugar, and lemons and mix well to dissolve the sugar thoroughly.

Add more water to fill the jar just two inches below the rim. Cover tightly and let the juice ferment for 2 days if you prefer it sweet, 3 days if you want it tangy. Transfer to cold storage and chill for 30 minutes before serving.
*Mouthwatering!*

# Kombucha

*This sweet tea is practically overloaded with good bacteria!*

## What You Need:
This recipe calls for 1 cup of raw honey, 13 cups of filtered water, 5 teaspoons of loose-leaf black tea, 1 cup of finished plain kombucha, and 1 piece of its supplementary scoby ( from your favorite organic food store).

## How to Make:
Separate 3 cups from the filtered water supply and bring to a boil. Next, add the sugar and let it dissolve before removing the solution from heat. Toss in the loose black tea leaves to soak while the sugar-water solution cools down.

Once your sweet tea is done, strain and pour it into a 1-gallon fermenting jar. Remove the tea leaves and add in the finished kombucha, scoby, and the remaining 10 cups of water. Let the solution ferment in a warm, dark place for 1 week. Transfer your kombucha to a covered glass jar (with at least 1 inch of space below the rim) and allow it to undergo further fermentation for 2 days, after which it can be placed in cold storage for up to 3 months.
*Enjoy!*

# Cultured Orange Juice

*This beverage puts a refreshing spin on your childhood favorite!*

**What You Need:**
For this recipe, you will need 3 cups of fresh squeezed orange juice, 1 cup of filtered water, and 2 tablespoons of whey.

**How to Make:**
In a 1-quart fermenting jar, pour in the orange juice, filtered water, and whey. Mix the solution well by covering the jar tightly and then giving it a good shake. Let it stand at room temperature for 2 days to ferment, after which it should be transferred immediately to your refrigerator. *Yay!*

# Chapter 5 Recipes for Fermented Desserts

## Fruity Kefir Ice Pops

*These ice pops look so adorable that you'll almost regret eating them!*

### What You Need:
This simple recipe calls for water kefir and 2 cups worth of various fruits: pineapple chunks, halved berries, chopped grapes, and mango slices. And that's it!

### How to Make:
Combine the assorted fruits in a large mixing bowl. Fill your ice pop molds with the mixed fruits, leaving some space that's about ¼ of the way.

Pour water kefir into the fruit-filled molds, and then freeze for 8-10 hours.    It is best to let the ice pops stand at room temperature for about 5 minutes before serving them.

*Delicious!*

# Heavenly Crème Fraiche

*Thoroughly rich and creamy and brimming with enzymes and minerals, this will serve as a satisfyingly delicious way to top off your desserts!*

**What You Need:**
This recipe calls for cream – whipped, half-and-half, or raw – whatever suits your taste is just fine. Whipped cream will give you the thickest crème fraiche you can possibly make; raw cream will give you one with a thinner consistency; and half-and-half should do if you like your crème fraiche with just the right amount of thickness that suits most people. Just keep in mind that ultra-high temperature (UHT) cream has no business being used in this recipe due to the inconsistent texture it yields when it undergoes fermentation.

The other necessity for this recipe is your starter culture. You can buy one that is specifically used to make crème fraiche. Just store it in the freezer until you are ready to whip up a mean crème fraiche.

**How to Make:**
You can start by warming the cream of your choice ever so slightly to 86°F before adding in the crème fraiche starter culture. Stir for about 15 seconds, transfer to a fermenting quart jar, and cover. Look for a warm spot that hovers between 72°F and 77°F and place the Mason jar in that

spot until the crème fraiche inside thickens, which usually happens after 12 to 18 hours.

If you want it thicker, simply let the crème fraiche pass through a clean tea towel. Let the resulting mixture set by putting the jar's cover back on and placing it in the refrigerator for 6 hours or more. This will serve to cool your crème fraiche as well as stop the fermentation process. As long stays refrigerated, this recipe should let your crème fraiche keep for up to a week.

*Delicious!*

## Super Creamy Vanilla Ice Cream

*This is not your usual vanilla ice cream!*

### What You Need:
For this recipe, you will need 1 cup of fresh cream, 1 ½ cups of half-and-half, 1 tablespoon of vanilla, ¼ teaspoon salt, 1 cup of crème fraiche, and 2 teaspoons of lemon juices.

### How to Make:
Combine the fresh cream, half-and-half, crème fraiche, and lemon juice in a large mixing bowl. Mix well, add the salt and vanilla, and whisk until the mixture becomes frothy. Let the mixture chill in the refrigerator for about 1 hour, after which it can be processed in your ice cream maker. Transfer your vanilla ice cream in a tightly covered container and keep in the freezer.

# Strawberry and Peaches Frozen Yogurt

*Here's a refreshingly tart spin on good old yogurt!*

**What You Need:**
For this recipe, you will need 4 cups of frozen peach chunks, ½ cup of plain yogurt, frozen slices of 5 large strawberries, 1 tablespoon of lemon juice, and 3 tablespoons of honey.

**How to Make:**
Place all ingredients in a blender and process until everything turns out creamy and smooth. You may serve your frozen yogurt immediately, or you may store it in a lidded container to keep in the freezer for no more than a month.
*Sweet!*

# Conclusion

Thank you again for downloading this book!
I hope this book was able to help you to become convinced that fermenting your own food does not have to be an intimidating task and that is actually simple and easy to do.

The next step is to not only enjoy eating fermented food and take advantage of its benefits to your health, but to also share your newfound passion and knowledge to friends and loved ones. It's a great way of spreading goodness to the world in more ways than one!

Finally, if you enjoyed this book, then I'd like to ask you for a favor. Would you be kind enough to leave a review for this book on Amazon? It'd be greatly appreciated!
Click here to leave a review for this book on Amazon!

Thank you and good luck!

# Bonus Content

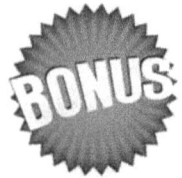

**As a token of our appreciation Grand Reveur Publications would like to give you access to our exclusive bonus content (including free eBooks!).**

*Exclusive pre-release access to our latest eBooks Free Grand Reveur eBooks during promotional periods.*

*A method ANYONE can use to publish their own book and make passive income.*

To receive Bonus Content visit the following page:

***https://ignorelimits.leadpages.net/grandreveurpublications/***

As this is a limited time offer it would be a shame to miss out, I recommend grabbing these bonuses before reading on.

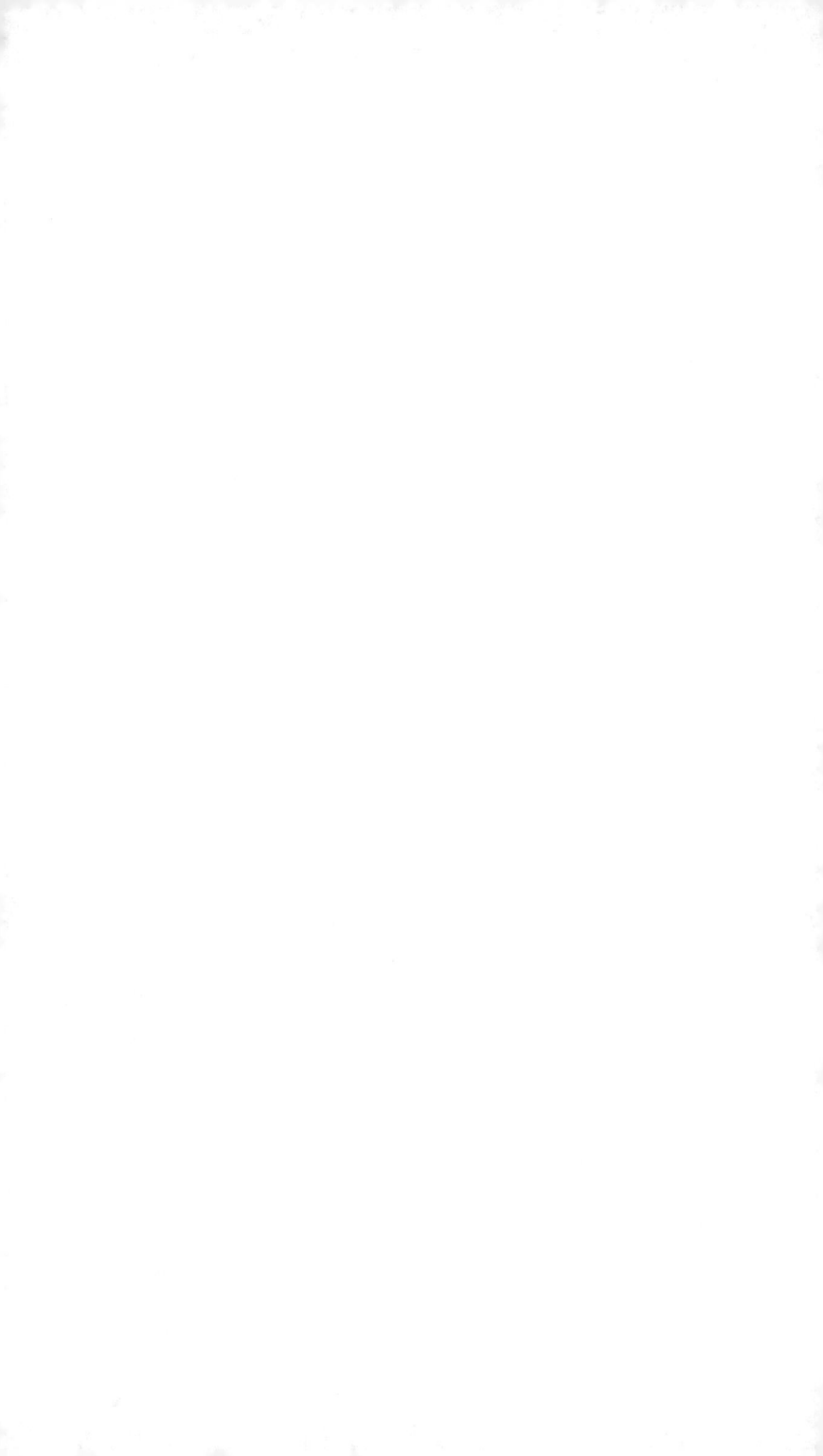

# Fermentation

## *Fermentation for Beginners, Fermentation Recipes rich in Probiotics, Enzymes, Vitamins, Minerals - LEARN To Ferment Foods Now*